Neo-Medrol Guide

Understanding the Usage, Benefits, and Precautions for Effective Skin Ailments Treatment with Neo-Medrol

EMILY JOHNSON

**PLEASE BE INFORMED
THAT THIS IS A BOOK**

All rights reserved.
Copyright © Emily Johnson, 2024

No part of this publication may be reproduced, distributed, or transmitted in any form or by any means, including photocopying, recording, or other electronic or mechanical methods, without the prior written permission of the publisher, except in the case of brief quotations embodied in critical reviews and certain other noncommercial uses permitted by copyright law.

The information in this book is for educational purposes only and is not medical advice. The author has made every effort to provide accurate and up-to-date information about the topic, but it should not replace professional medical guidance. Consult with a qualified healthcare provider before starting or stopping any medication, including Neo-Medrol. Only a healthcare professional can provide personalized advice based on your health needs. The author and publisher are not responsible for any adverse effects from using this information.

Contents

Chapter 1..9
Introduction to Neo Medrol........................ 9
   Understanding Neomycin and Medrysone....... 12
   Common Conditions Treated with Neo Medrol... 15

Chapter 2.. 22
How to Use Neo Medrol Safely.................. 22
   Proper Application Techniques........................ 23
   Dosage and Frequency: What You Need to Know 27
   Avoiding Overuse: Why Following Instructions Matters............30

Chapter 3.. 35
Understanding the Side Effects.................. 35
   Common Side Effects: What to Expect.............36
   Rare but Serious Reactions...............................39
   Managing Mild Irritations and When to Seek Medical Help............42

Chapter 4.. 48
Precautions and Warnings.....................48

Who Should Not Use Neo Medrol?................... 49
Drug Interactions and Allergies........................52

Chapter 5.. 60
Tips for Maximizing the Benefits.............. 60
Combining Neo Medrol with Other Treatments.. 61
Lifestyle Tips to Support Skin Healing.............65
How to Prevent the Recurrence of Skin Issues 68

Chapter 6...73
20 Frequently Asked Questions About Neo Medrol.. 73

Chapter 7.. 86
Storage and Expiry Information............... 86
Proper Storage to Maintain Effectiveness........ 87

Conclusion.. 97

Chapter 1

Introduction to Neo Medrol

Neo Medrol is a topical medication that plays a vital role in treating various skin conditions marked by inflammation and potential infection. Its importance in the dermatology field cannot be overstated, as it has helped many people with chronic or acute skin conditions find relief. But what exactly is Neo Medrol, and what makes it so effective? To understand its value, we need to look closely at its composition, how it works, and why it's prescribed.

Neo Medrol combines two potent ingredients: neomycin, an antibiotic, and medrysone, a corticosteroid. This duo creates a powerful synergy that tackles both the inflammation often present in skin disorders and any bacterial infections that may accompany it. People often use Neo Medrol for conditions like eczema, dermatitis, or even more severe inflammatory skin diseases where secondary infections are a concern. This versatility is one of the reasons Neo Medrol is frequently prescribed by dermatologists.

The idea behind combining these two active ingredients is simple but effective. Skin issues are often multifaceted, meaning they might not just be a case of irritation but also carry a risk of bacterial infections. Neo Medrol addresses both problems in one product, making it a comprehensive treatment option for many people.

For anyone who has experienced skin issues like eczema or an allergic reaction, the irritation can feel unbearable. It can disrupt your daily life and, in some cases, impact your confidence. Neo Medrol is designed to soothe the skin, reducing swelling, redness, and irritation, while also fighting off infections that might make the condition worse. Its dual-action formula brings rapid relief, allowing individuals to go about their lives with less discomfort.

Understanding Neomycin and Medrysone

The real beauty of Neo Medrol lies in its two primary components: neomycin and medrysone. These two ingredients complement each other, making the treatment both potent and safe when used correctly.

Neomycin is a well-known antibiotic, effective against a broad spectrum of bacteria that can cause skin infections. Bacteria thrive in the warmth and moisture of inflamed skin, and they can quickly turn a simple irritation into something much more serious. Neomycin works by inhibiting bacterial growth, thus preventing infection and allowing the skin to heal properly. Its presence in Neo Medrol ensures that the skin is not only healing from inflammation but also protected from external bacterial threats.

Medrysone, on the other hand, is a corticosteroid. Steroids like Medrysone work by reducing inflammation. When your body reacts to something harmful—like allergens or irritants—it triggers an inflammatory response. While this is a natural defense mechanism, in many cases, the inflammation becomes a problem in itself, leading to swelling, redness, and pain. Medrysone helps calm this response, bringing much-needed relief to the affected skin. It also works to reduce itching, which can be one of the most frustrating symptoms of skin conditions. Itchiness often leads to scratching, which can further damage the skin and make infections more likely. By reducing itching, medrysone indirectly protects the skin from further harm.

Together, neomycin and medrysone create a medication that treats both the cause and symptoms of many skin conditions. Neomycin targets bacterial infections, while Medrysone reduces inflammation and the discomfort that comes with it. This dual approach is what makes Neo Medrol such an effective treatment for a wide range of skin issues.

Common Conditions Treated with Neo Medrol

Neo Medrol is a versatile treatment, prescribed for some different skin conditions. Some of the most common conditions treated with Neo Medrol include eczema, dermatitis, psoriasis, and seborrheic dermatitis, among others. Each of these conditions shares one common characteristic: inflammation. However, they differ in the triggers and additional complications, which is why having a medication that addresses both infection and inflammation is so valuable.

1. **Eczema**: One of the most prevalent conditions treated with Neo Medrol is eczema, also known as atopic dermatitis.

Eczema is a chronic condition where patches of skin become inflamed, itchy, and cracked. In severe cases, these patches can also ooze fluid, leading to bacterial infections. Because eczema compromises the skin's barrier, it becomes more susceptible to infections. The neomycin in Neo Medrol helps prevent these infections, while Medrysone reduces the itching and inflammation that makes eczema so unbearable. For someone with eczema, relief can feel like a lifeline, allowing them to stop scratching and let their skin heal.

2. **Contact Dermatitis**: Contact dermatitis occurs when the skin reacts to a substance it comes into contact with. This might be a harsh chemical, an allergen like poison ivy, or even certain metals in jewelry. The result

is red, inflamed skin that can be extremely uncomfortable. Neo Medrol helps by calming the immune response that leads to inflammation, while also guarding against infections that may develop if the skin becomes damaged. Its use in contact dermatitis is particularly helpful for those who experience severe allergic reactions that might lead to blisters or open sores.

3. **Seborrheic Dermatitis**: Seborrheic dermatitis is another condition commonly treated with Neo Medrol. This condition typically affects areas of the body with a high density of oil glands, such as the scalp, face, and upper chest. It leads to scaly patches, red skin, and stubborn dandruff. The inflammation is the main problem, but because the condition affects areas that are

prone to moisture, there's also a heightened risk of bacterial or fungal infections. Neo Medrol helps in two ways: by reducing inflammation and by keeping infections at bay.

4. **Psoriasis**: Psoriasis is a chronic autoimmune condition where the skin cells multiply faster than usual, causing scales and red patches. These patches are often itchy and painful, and because the skin is constantly inflamed, there's a risk of secondary infections. Neo Medrol is not typically a first-line treatment for psoriasis, but it is sometimes prescribed in cases where infections complicate the condition. By reducing both inflammation and preventing infections, it offers a

two-pronged approach to managing the symptoms.

5. **Intertrigo**: Intertrigo is a rash that occurs in skin folds, such as under the breasts, in the groin area, or between the thighs. It happens when moisture and friction irritate the skin, leading to inflammation and, in some cases, infections. Because it often occurs in areas where sweat accumulates, infections are a major concern. Neo Medrol can be an excellent treatment option because it tackles both the irritation and the infection risk. Its soothing properties can reduce the pain and discomfort associated with intertrigo, while its antibacterial component ensures that the rash doesn't become a more serious infection.

6. **Bacterial Skin Infections**: In addition to treating inflammatory skin conditions, Neo Medrol is also sometimes used to treat simple bacterial infections. This can be particularly useful in cases where an infection develops alongside an existing skin condition, or when a minor injury, such as a cut or abrasion, becomes infected. Neomycin helps eliminate the bacteria causing the infection, while medrysone reduces the swelling and discomfort.

In each of these conditions, Neo Medrol's combination of neomycin and medrysone offers relief not just from the symptoms, but also from potential complications like infections. Whether someone is dealing with a chronic skin condition like eczema or a more acute issue like contact dermatitis, the dual-action formula of Neo Medrol helps ensure that they can find relief from inflammation and protect against infections.

Neo Medrol stands out as an effective and reliable treatment for a wide range of skin conditions. By combining the power of neomycin and medrysone, it addresses both the inflammation and infection risks that often accompany skin issues. For those struggling with chronic skin conditions or acute reactions, Neo Medrol offers a comprehensive solution that not only treats the symptoms but also promotes healing and prevents complications.

Chapter 2

How to Use Neo Medrol Safely

Using medications like Neo Medrol safely and effectively requires not only understanding how they work but also knowing how to apply them correctly and when to stop or start using them. Topical medications like Neo Medrol are powerful tools, and when used properly, they can provide tremendous relief from a variety of skin conditions. However, it's crucial to use them as directed to avoid complications or diminish their effectiveness. In this section, we'll discuss proper application techniques, dosage and frequency, and why it's essential to avoid overuse.

Proper Application Techniques

Applying Neo Medrol may seem straightforward, but there are important steps that can ensure you're getting the most benefit from the treatment while minimizing risks. One of the first things to remember is that clean skin is key. Applying the medication to unclean skin can trap dirt and bacteria, possibly making the condition worse or causing a new infection.

Before using Neo Medrol, wash the affected area gently with soap and water. This helps remove any dirt, oils, or bacteria from the skin's surface, ensuring that the medication can be fully absorbed. After washing, make sure the skin is completely dry before applying the medication. This is important because applying Neo Medrol to wet skin can dilute the medication or spread it to areas where it's not needed, leading to potential side effects like irritation or weakening of the skin barrier.

When you're ready to apply Neo Medrol, use clean hands or a sterile applicator to avoid contaminating the medication or the affected area. A small amount of the ointment should be enough—just enough to cover the area with a thin layer. More is not better in this case, and overapplying the medication can increase the risk of side effects without improving the treatment results.

It's also a good idea to avoid rubbing the medication in too aggressively. Gently patting or lightly spreading the ointment is usually enough. Rubbing too hard can further irritate the already sensitive skin or cause the medication to wear off too quickly.

Another key point is to avoid applying Neo Medrol to large areas of the body unless specifically instructed by your healthcare provider. This is because the skin absorbs corticosteroids like medrysone, and applying them to larger areas increases the risk of systemic side effects. Similarly, Neo Medrol should not be applied to broken or severely damaged skin unless a doctor has advised you to do so. In some cases, an open wound can absorb too much of the medication, leading to complications.

If you're treating an area that's covered by clothing, try to allow the medication to absorb into the skin before covering it. Covering the treated area immediately after application can trap moisture and increase the likelihood of irritation or secondary infections. If your doctor has instructed you to use a bandage or wrap over the treated area, be sure to follow those instructions carefully, as there are cases where covering the treated skin can help the medication work more effectively.

Finally, wash your hands thoroughly after applying the medication, especially if you're treating an area that's prone to infection or irritation. This prevents any accidental transfer of the medication to other parts of your body or other people.

Dosage and Frequency: What You Need to Know

Understanding the correct dosage and frequency is just as important as knowing how to apply NeoMedrol. Because it's a powerful topical medication, following the prescribed dosage is crucial to avoid complications or side effects, especially if you're using it for an extended period.

Neo Medrol is typically applied once or twice a day, depending on the severity of the condition and the specific instructions from your healthcare provider. It's important to follow these instructions closely, as applying it more frequently than recommended won't speed up the healing process and may worsen the side effects. If you're using it twice daily, try to space the applications out evenly, such as once in the morning and once in the evening, to maintain consistent levels of the medication on the skin.

Over-the-counter products often allow a little more flexibility, but prescription medications like Neo Medrol require precise adherence to your doctor's recommendations. If you're unsure about how often to apply it, always check with your healthcare provider rather than guessing or applying it more frequently than suggested.

In some cases, your doctor may recommend a gradual reduction in the frequency of use, especially if you've been using Neo Medrol for an extended period. This helps to prevent withdrawal symptoms or a flare-up of the skin condition, a phenomenon known as the "rebound effect." The body can become dependent on the corticosteroid in the medication, and stopping it abruptly can cause the skin to react negatively, with symptoms like increased redness, itching, or swelling.

Another important point is to avoid skipping doses. If you miss an application, apply it as soon as you remember. However, if it's almost time for your next dose, skip the missed application and continue with your regular schedule. Doubling up on doses to make up for missed ones can lead to overuse, increasing the risk of side effects.

For those who are using Neo Medrol on an ongoing basis, it's essential to have regular check-ins with your healthcare provider. This ensures that the medication is still necessary and that you're not experiencing any long-term side effects. In some cases, your doctor may recommend taking a break from the medication or switching to a milder treatment once your symptoms are under control.

Avoiding Overuse: Why Following Instructions Matters

One of the most common mistakes people make with topical medications like Neo Medrol is overuse. It's easy to think that applying more frequently or using larger amounts of the medication will help the condition heal faster, but this is a dangerous misconception.

Neo Medrol contains a corticosteroid, which is very effective at reducing inflammation but can also have significant side effects if used improperly. Overuse of corticosteroids can lead to skin thinning (atrophy), stretch marks, and even systemic effects if too much of the medication is absorbed into the bloodstream. Skin thinning, in particular, is a concern with prolonged or excessive use. When the skin becomes too thin, it's more prone to injury, infections, and bruising, making it even harder for the skin to heal.

In addition to skin thinning, overusing Neo Medrol can cause other issues, such as increased hair growth in the treated area, discoloration of the skin, and acne-like eruptions. These side effects can be distressing, especially for people who are already dealing with sensitive or damaged skin.

Moreover, overusing the neomycin component of Neo Medrol can lead to antibiotic resistance. This happens when bacteria on your skin become resistant to the antibiotic, making it less effective over time. Antibiotic resistance is a serious global health concern, and it can make future infections more difficult to treat. It's important to use Neo Medrol only as prescribed to avoid contributing to this issue.

Another risk of overuse is the possibility of systemic side effects. Although rare with topical medications, when corticosteroids are absorbed in large amounts, they can affect the entire body. This can lead to side effects such as weight gain, high blood pressure, and changes in blood sugar levels. While these effects are uncommon, they're more likely if you're applying the medication to large areas of the body or using it for an extended period without medical supervision.

To avoid overuse, it's crucial to follow your healthcare provider's instructions carefully. Use the smallest amount of medication necessary to cover the affected area and stick to the recommended application frequency. If you feel that the medication isn't working as quickly as you'd like, resist the temptation to increase the dose on your own. Instead, consult your doctor, who may adjust your treatment plan if necessary.

Using Neo Medrol safely requires attention to detail and adherence to medical advice. By applying the medication correctly, following the prescribed dosage and frequency, and avoiding overuse, you can maximize the benefits of Neo Medrol while minimizing the risks. Proper usage not only helps your skin heal but also ensures that you can continue using this effective treatment without complications.

Chapter 3

Understanding the Side Effects

Like any medication, Neo Mcdrol, while effective in treating various skin conditions, can come with its share of side effects. Being aware of what to expect can help reduce the anxiety that often comes with using a new medication and empower you to manage any issues that may arise. Some side effects are common and expected, while others are more serious but fortunately rare. It is also crucial to know how to manage mild irritations and when it's time to seek medical advice.

Common Side Effects: What to Expect

Neo Medrol is a combination of two active ingredients—neomycin, an antibiotic, and medrysone, a corticosteroid. These components work together to reduce inflammation and fight bacterial infections. While highly effective, both neomycin and medrysone can cause side effects, especially when used for extended periods or on sensitive skin.

One of the most common side effects users report is mild irritation at the application site. This can manifest as slight redness, a mild burning sensation, or itching. This kind of irritation is typically temporary, occurring shortly after application and usually subsiding within a few hours. It can be unsettling at first, especially if your skin is already inflamed, but it's often a sign that the medication is beginning to work by stimulating the affected area.

Skin dryness is another frequent side effect. Corticosteroids, like Medrysone, can reduce the natural oils in the skin, leading to patches of dryness. For some, this may feel like tight or flaky skin after applying the medication. This side effect can be managed by applying a gentle, fragrance-free moisturizer to the unaffected areas, but it's important to avoid applying moisturizers directly on the area where Neo Medrol is used unless advised by a healthcare provider.

Increased sensitivity to sunlight is also common. Topical medications, particularly those containing corticosteroids, can make the skin more vulnerable to sun damage. This means that after applying Neo Medrol, your skin may be more prone to sunburn, even with minimal sun exposure. To minimize this risk, it's a good idea to wear protective clothing or apply sunscreen to areas exposed to the sun, but not over the medication itself. Staying out of direct sunlight while using Neo Medrol is the safest option if possible.

Another side effect that some people experience is changes in skin appearance. For example, there may be temporary lightening or darkening of the skin where the medication is applied. This happens because corticosteroids can affect the pigment cells in the skin, especially when used for prolonged periods or over large areas. In most cases, these changes are temporary and will resolve after discontinuing the medication.

Rare but Serious Reactions

While most side effects of Neo Medrol are mild, it's important to be aware of rare but serious reactions that may require immediate medical attention. These side effects are uncommon but can be severe if they occur.

One of the most serious side effects is an allergic reaction to neomycin. Some people may develop contact dermatitis, a type of skin rash that occurs as a reaction to the antibiotic component. Signs of an allergic reaction include intense redness, swelling, itching, or a rash that worsens despite using the medication. In some cases, blisters or oozing sores may develop. If you suspect an allergic reaction, it's important to stop using the medication immediately and contact your healthcare provider for advice. They may recommend an alternative treatment or prescribe medication to manage the allergic response.

Another rare but concerning side effect is systemic absorption of the corticosteroid. While Neo Medrol is a topical medication intended to act locally on the skin, small amounts of medrysone can be absorbed into the bloodstream, particularly if the medication is used on large areas of the skin or for prolonged periods. This can lead to systemic side effects similar to those seen with oral corticosteroids, such as weight gain, mood changes, or increased blood pressure. In extremely rare cases, long-term use of topical corticosteroids can lead to adrenal suppression, a condition where the body's adrenal glands reduce their natural production of cortisol. This can cause symptoms like fatigue, muscle weakness, or dizziness, especially if the medication is stopped suddenly. Fortunately, these side effects are highly uncommon with proper use, but it's important to follow your healthcare provider's instructions closely and use the lowest effective dose for the shortest time possible.

Another serious reaction to be aware of is the development of secondary infections. While Neo Medrol contains an antibiotic, overuse or improper use can disrupt the balance of bacteria on your skin, potentially leading to fungal or other bacterial infections. If you notice increased redness, swelling, pus, or worsening of the condition after starting treatment, it could indicate an infection. Seek medical advice right away to determine the best course of action.

Managing Mild Irritations and When to Seek Medical Help

For most users, the side effects of Neo Medrol will be mild and easily manageable. Understanding how to address these minor irritations can help you continue treatment without interruption.

If you experience mild redness, itching, or dryness after applying Neo Medrol, there are several steps you can take to alleviate these symptoms. First, try applying the medication less frequently, especially if you're using it more than once a day. Giving your skin time to rest between applications may reduce irritation. Additionally, consider applying a cool compress to the affected area for a few minutes after applying the medication. This can help soothe the skin and reduce inflammation, making the treatment more comfortable.

If dryness is a persistent issue, using a gentle moisturizer can be helpful. Look for products that are labeled "non-comedogenic" and free from fragrances or dyes, as these are less likely to irritate sensitive skin. Apply the moisturizer to surrounding areas, but avoid applying it directly over the medication unless otherwise advised by your healthcare provider.

Sun sensitivity can also be managed by wearing protective clothing and staying out of direct sunlight, especially during peak hours. If you need to be outside, wearing a broad-spectrum sunscreen with an SPF of 30 or higher can provide additional protection. However, be sure not to apply sunscreen directly over the medicated area unless recommended by your doctor.

If you experience more severe side effects, it's essential to know when to seek medical help. If you notice signs of an allergic reaction, such as hives, intense itching, or swelling, discontinue the medication immediately and contact your healthcare provider. In some cases, you may need a different medication or additional treatment to manage the allergic response.

If the condition being treated with Neo Medrol worsens or doesn't improve after several days of use, consult your doctor. The underlying condition may require a different treatment approach, or a secondary infection has developed. Similarly, if you notice any unusual symptoms like excessive weight gain, mood changes, or fatigue, which could indicate systemic absorption of the medication, it's important to contact your healthcare provider immediately.

In rare cases, a sudden worsening of the skin condition after stopping Neo Medrol could indicate a rebound effect, where the skin becomes dependent on the corticosteroid. If this happens, consult your doctor about how to taper off the medication gradually to avoid withdrawal symptoms.

In summary, understanding the potential side effects of Neo Medrol and knowing how to manage them can help you get the most out of your treatment while minimizing discomfort. Most side effects are mild and manageable, but being aware of the more serious reactions and knowing when to seek help ensures that you can use NeoMedrol safely and effectively. By following your healthcare provider's instructions and keeping an open line of communication, you can address any concerns promptly and confidently manage your treatment.

Chapter 4

Precautions and Warnings

When using any medication, especially one that combines both an antibiotic and a corticosteroid like Neo Medrol, it is important to be aware of specific precautions and warnings to ensure safe and effective treatment. Neo Medrol can be a powerful solution for managing skin infections and inflammation, but it's not suitable for everyone, and there are particular areas of the body where special care must be taken. By understanding who should avoid using this medication, how it interacts with other drugs, and the precautions necessary when applying it to sensitive areas like the face or eyes, users can make more informed decisions about their treatment.

Who Should Not Use Neo Medrol?

While Neo Medrol is effective for many people, certain conditions and factors can make it inappropriate or risky for some individuals. One of the most important precautions is to avoid using Neo Medrol if you have a known allergy to either of its active ingredients—neomycin or medrysone. Allergic reactions to neomycin, in particular, are not uncommon, and symptoms can range from mild irritation to severe skin reactions. If you have a history of allergic contact dermatitis or other skin sensitivities, especially to antibiotics or steroids, it's crucial to inform your doctor before starting treatment with Neo Medrol.

Another group of people who should be cautious about using Neo Medrol includes those with viral, fungal, or tubercular skin infections. The corticosteroid component (medrysone) works by suppressing inflammation and the immune response, which can be beneficial in reducing swelling and irritation. However, it also reduces the body's ability to fight off infections, making it potentially dangerous to use on skin conditions caused by viruses (like herpes simplex), fungi (such as athlete's foot), or tuberculosis. In these cases, Neo Medrol could worsen the infection or mask symptoms, leading to complications. If you suspect your skin condition is caused by a virus or fungus, consult your healthcare provider for an alternative treatment.

Additionally, individuals with a history of severe skin thinning or conditions like eczema and psoriasis should be cautious. Long-term or excessive use of corticosteroids can lead to thinning of the skin, which may aggravate certain conditions. While Neo Medrol may be prescribed for short-term use in these cases, it's important to follow the dosage and application instructions carefully and avoid prolonged use. If you have a chronic skin condition, your doctor may recommend monitoring the treatment more closely to minimize the risk of complications.

Pregnant and breastfeeding women should also take special care. Although there is limited data on the effects of Neo Medrol during pregnancy, corticosteroids, and antibiotics can sometimes pose risks to fetal development or pass into breast milk. If you are pregnant or nursing, it's essential to consult with your healthcare provider before using Neo Medrol to weigh the potential benefits and risks.

Drug Interactions and Allergies

Like any medication, Neo Medrol can interact with other drugs or exacerbate existing allergies, leading to adverse reactions. One of the most common concerns when it comes to drug interactions involves other topical treatments or medications being used in the same area.

For instance, if you're already using another topical antibiotic, antifungal cream, or steroid, applying Neo Medrol in addition could increase the risk of irritation or weaken the effectiveness of one or both treatments. Be sure to inform your doctor about all the medications you are using, both over-the-counter and prescription, so they can determine if Neo Medrol is suitable.

One interaction worth noting is with other corticosteroid medications. If you're taking oral or injectable steroids for other conditions, using a topical corticosteroid like Neo Medrol in large amounts could increase the overall steroid load on your body. This could potentially lead to systemic side effects, such as hormonal imbalances, weight gain, or adrenal suppression. Always check with your healthcare provider before combining multiple steroid-based treatments to avoid these complications.

Allergic reactions are also a concern, particularly for people with sensitivities to antibiotics in the aminoglycoside family, which includes neomycin. Allergies to neomycin can manifest as redness, itching, rash, or even blistering and oozing at the application site. If you've had allergic reactions to neomycin or similar antibiotics in the past, it's important to let your doctor know before using Neo Medrol. In some cases, your doctor may recommend a patch test—a small application of the medication on a small area of skin—to check for allergic reactions before proceeding with full treatment.

Additionally, people who have a history of severe allergies or asthma should use caution with Neo Medrol, as the immune-suppressing effects of corticosteroids can sometimes trigger adverse reactions. Though rare, some individuals with preexisting allergies may experience systemic allergic responses, such as difficulty breathing, hives, or swelling after using topical corticosteroids. If you experience any signs of a serious allergic reaction, such as difficulty breathing, swelling of the face or throat, or severe rash, seek medical attention immediately.

Using Neo Medrol on Sensitive Areas: Face, Eyes, and Mucous Membranes

One of the key precautions when using Neo Medrol is to be cautious about where you apply it. The skin on certain areas of the body, such as the face, around the eyes, and near mucous membranes (like inside the mouth or nose), is much more sensitive and prone to irritation than other areas. Using Neo Medrol on these delicate areas requires extra care to avoid complications.

The face, in particular, is a common area where people may be tempted to apply Neo Medrol due to the prevalence of conditions like acne or rosacea. While Neo Medrol can reduce inflammation and bacterial infection, using corticosteroids on the face, especially for extended periods, can lead to thinning of the skin, the development of small red or purple spots (caused by weakened blood vessels), and even acne-like breakouts. If your doctor has prescribed Neo Medrol for use on the face, it's important to apply it sparingly and only for the prescribed duration. Be mindful of any changes in skin texture or color and report them to your healthcare provider if they occur.

The area around the eyes is especially vulnerable to corticosteroids. Using Neo Medrol too close to the eyes can lead to an increased risk of glaucoma, cataracts, or other eye problems, as the medication may be absorbed into the eye through the thin skin around it. It's critical to avoid getting the medication in your eyes, and if you accidentally do, rinse thoroughly with water and seek medical advice. If you have a condition affecting the skin around your eyes, your healthcare provider may recommend alternative treatments specifically designed for use in this sensitive area.

Mucous membranes, such as the inside of the mouth, nose, or genital area, are also particularly susceptible to irritation from medications like Neo Medrol. Applying this medication to mucous membranes can lead to burning, stinging, or even damage to the tissue. If your skin condition involves these areas, it's important to discuss alternative treatments with your doctor, as Neo Medrol is not typically recommended for use on mucous membranes.

In summary, understanding the precautions and warnings associated with Neo Medrol is essential for using the medication safely and effectively. While this medication can offer significant relief for bacterial infections and inflammation, it is not suitable for everyone, and specific considerations must be taken into account based on your medical history, current medications, and the area of application. By discussing any concerns with your healthcare provider and following the prescribed guidelines, you can reduce the risk of side effects and ensure the best possible outcome from your treatment.

Chapter 5

Tips for Maximizing the Benefits

When using a medication like Neo Medrol, which combines both antibiotic and corticosteroid properties, it's essential to optimize its use for the best possible results. Neo Medrol can effectively treat various skin conditions, but understanding how to integrate it with other treatments, support your body through lifestyle changes, and prevent future flare-ups will help maximize its benefits. The following tips are aimed at ensuring you get the most from your treatment, while also focusing on long-term skin health and prevention of recurring issues.

Combining Neo Medrol with Other Treatments

One of the best ways to maximize the benefits of Neo Medrol is to combine it, where appropriate, with other treatments. Since Neo Medrol targets both bacterial infections and inflammation, it may not address all aspects of a skin condition. In some cases, integrating additional treatments can offer a more comprehensive solution.

For example, if your skin condition includes a fungal component (such as a mixed bacterial and fungal infection), your doctor might recommend using an antifungal cream alongside Neo Medrol. By addressing both the bacterial and fungal aspects simultaneously, the treatment becomes more effective, reducing the likelihood of incomplete healing or recurrence. It's crucial, however, to avoid self-prescribing other treatments without consulting your healthcare provider. Certain medications might interact negatively with Neo Medrol, and a healthcare professional will guide you on safe combinations.

Similarly, for individuals dealing with chronic inflammatory skin conditions like eczema or psoriasis, moisturizing routines can be a vital complement to Neo Medrol. Corticosteroids like Medrysone can help reduce inflammation, but they may also dry out the skin over time. Adding a high-quality, fragrance-free moisturizer to your daily routine can help restore the skin's natural barrier and reduce itching and irritation. For some, doctors may also recommend the use of hydrating ointments or emollients in conjunction with Neo Medrol to lock in moisture and further support healing.

In more severe cases, Neo Medrol may be part of a broader treatment plan that includes oral medications. For conditions like severe allergic reactions or widespread skin infections, oral antibiotics or oral corticosteroids might be prescribed alongside the topical application of Neo Medrol. This combined approach can target the problem both at the surface and systemically, ensuring a more thorough and efficient recovery.

Additionally, if your skin condition stems from an underlying medical issue, such as a hormonal imbalance or immune system disorder, your doctor might suggest treatments aimed at addressing the root cause. By tackling the condition at its source, you reduce the risk of persistent or recurring skin problems and improve the overall outcome of your Neo Medrol treatment.

Lifestyle Tips to Support Skin Healing

Beyond medication, lifestyle habits play a significant role in how well your skin heals and how effectively Neo Medrol works. One of the simplest but most effective things you can do to support healing is to maintain good skin hygiene. Keeping the affected area clean and free from dirt, oils, and bacteria can enhance the action of the medication. However, it's essential to balance cleanliness with gentleness—over-scrubbing or using harsh soaps can further irritate inflamed skin. Opt for mild, hypoallergenic cleansers, and avoid exfoliating the treated area unless directed by your doctor.

Diet can also influence the healing process. Proper nutrition supports the body's natural healing mechanisms and can help reduce inflammation. Foods rich in antioxidants, such as berries, leafy greens, and nuts, can support skin repair by fighting free radicals and promoting collagen production. Omega-3 fatty acids, found in foods like salmon, flaxseed, and walnuts, are known to have anti-inflammatory properties and may help reduce skin irritation. Staying hydrated is equally important. Drinking enough water throughout the day helps keep the skin hydrated from within, which can aid in healing and reduce the dryness that sometimes accompanies corticosteroid use.

Stress management is another crucial aspect of skin health that is often overlooked.

Chronic stress can exacerbate skin conditions, triggering flare-ups or worsening symptoms. If you're dealing with a long-term skin issue like eczema or psoriasis, stress reduction techniques such as meditation, deep breathing exercises, or regular physical activity may help improve your condition. Incorporating mindfulness practices into your daily routine not only supports overall well-being but also enhances your skin's ability to recover and regenerate.

Sleep is equally vital in supporting skin health. During deep sleep, the body goes through a process of repair and regeneration, including the skin. Aim for 7-9 hours of restful sleep per night to give your skin the time it needs to heal properly. Poor sleep can impair the immune system and delay recovery, so establishing good sleep hygiene—such as keeping a regular sleep schedule and creating a calm bedtime environment—can be beneficial to your skin healing journey.

How to Prevent the Recurrence of Skin Issues

Once your skin condition has improved with the help of Neo Medrol, preventing recurrence becomes a top priority. For many people, skin conditions can be cyclical, flaring up in response to certain triggers or environmental factors. By identifying and managing these triggers, you can reduce the likelihood of future flare-ups.

One of the first steps in preventing recurrence is to continue following any maintenance treatment plan your doctor recommends. Even if your symptoms have cleared up, using Neo Medrol as directed for the full prescribed duration is essential to ensuring that the infection or inflammation doesn't return. Prematurely stopping the medication, even when symptoms improve, can lead to incomplete treatment and a quick recurrence of the condition.

Skin irritants are a common cause of recurring skin issues. Identifying potential irritants in your environment—whether they are soaps, lotions, household cleaners, or even certain fabrics—can help you avoid future flare-ups. For individuals prone to allergic reactions or dermatitis, switching to hypoallergenic, fragrance-free products may help keep the skin calm and free from irritation. In addition, if you have a known sensitivity to certain metals, chemicals, or plants, taking care to avoid contact with those substances can go a long way in preventing skin problems from coming back.

Sun exposure is another factor that can trigger flare-ups of certain skin conditions, especially for people with conditions like rosacea or lupus. Protecting your skin from UV damage by wearing sunscreen and protective clothing and seeking shade when outdoors can prevent sun-related irritation. If you are using Neo Medrol on sun-exposed areas, remember that corticosteroids can sometimes make the skin more sensitive to sunlight, so additional sun protection measures may be necessary.

Finally, maintaining a regular skincare routine that emphasizes prevention is key. Keeping the skin moisturized and protected helps reinforce the skin barrier, making it less vulnerable to infections or inflammatory responses. Using gentle, non-comedogenic products and avoiding harsh treatments like chemical peels or abrasive exfoliation can help preserve the skin's integrity and minimize the risk of recurrence.

Maximizing the benefits of Neo Medrol treatment involves a combination of safe and effective medication use, lifestyle adjustments, and proactive measures to prevent future skin issues. By working closely with your healthcare provider, integrating appropriate complementary treatments, and taking care of your skin through diet, stress management, and environmental precautions, you can achieve better results and support long-term skin health.

Chapter 6

20 Frequently Asked Questions About Neo Medrol

When it comes to using any medication, it's natural to have a lot of questions—whether you're curious about how it works, its side effects, or how it fits into your daily routine. Neo Medrol, a combination of neomycin and medrysone, is commonly prescribed for skin infections and inflammation, but patients often want to know more before starting treatment. Here, we answer 20 of the most frequently asked questions about Neo Medrol, providing insights that will help you make informed decisions and use the medication safely and effectively.

1. What is Neo Medrol used for?

Neo Medrol is a topical medication used to treat skin conditions that involve both infection and inflammation. It combines an antibiotic (neomycin) to fight bacterial infections and a corticosteroid (medrysone) to reduce swelling, redness, and irritation. It's commonly prescribed for conditions like infected eczema, dermatitis, and minor skin injuries that have become inflamed or infected.

2. How does Neo Medrol work?

Neo Medrol works by tackling two issues at once. Neomycin, the antibiotic, kills bacteria by preventing them from producing proteins they need to survive. Medrysone, the corticosteroid, reduces the body's inflammatory response, which helps decrease swelling, itching, and redness. Together, they help clear up infections and reduce irritation.

3. How should I apply Neo Medrol?

Neo Medrol should be applied as a thin layer to the affected area, typically two to four times a day, depending on your doctor's recommendation. Make sure the skin is clean and dry before applying the ointment. Gently massage it into the skin, but avoid rubbing too hard as this could further irritate the area.

4. Can I use Neo Medrol on my face?

Yes, Neo Medrol can be used on the face, but with caution. The skin on your face is more sensitive than other areas, so follow your doctor's instructions carefully. Avoid applying it near the eyes or on broken skin. If you're using it on your face for an extended period, regular follow-up with your healthcare provider is recommended to monitor for potential side effects like thinning of the skin.

5. How long does it take for Neo Medrol to work?
Most people begin to notice an improvement in their symptoms within a few days of starting NeoMedrol. The infection usually clears up within one to two weeks, but the exact timeline depends on the severity of the condition and how

consistently you apply the medication. If you don't see improvement after a week or if your symptoms worsen, consult your doctor.

6. Can I use Neo Medrol for a fungal infection?

No, Neo Medrol is not effective against fungal infections. It is designed to treat bacterial infections and reduce inflammation. If you suspect a fungal infection, you should speak with your doctor about antifungal treatment options, as using Neo Medrol on fungal infections may worsen the condition.

7. What should I do if I miss a dose?

If you forget to apply Neo Medrol, apply it as soon as you remember. However, if it's almost time for your next scheduled application, skip the missed dose and continue with your regular schedule. Do not double the amount to make up for the missed dose, as this can increase the risk of side effects.

8. **Can Neo Medrol be used on children?**

Yes, Neo Medrol can be prescribed to children, but it should be used with caution. Children's skin is more sensitive, and they are more likely to absorb corticosteroids into the bloodstream, which could lead to side effects. Always follow your pediatrician's instructions regarding the frequency and duration of use.

9. **Are there any side effects I should be aware of?**

Common side effects of Neo Medrol include mild skin irritation, redness, or itching at the application site. These effects are usually temporary and should resolve on their own. However, if you experience severe reactions like skin thinning, stretch marks, or increased sensitivity, stop using the medication and consult your doctor.

10. Can I use NeoMedrol if I'm pregnant or breastfeeding?

If you are pregnant or breastfeeding, it's important to discuss this with your healthcare provider before using Neo Medrol. While the medication is applied topically and the amount absorbed into the bloodstream is low, it's always better to be cautious when using any medication during pregnancy or while breastfeeding.

11. Can I apply Neo Medrol on open wounds?

No, Neo Medrol should not be applied to open or broken skin unless specifically directed by your doctor. Applying it to open wounds could increase the risk of absorbing the medication into the bloodstream or causing additional irritation.

12. Is Neo Medrol safe for long-term use?

Long-term use of Neo Medrol is not generally recommended because of the potential side effects of prolonged corticosteroid use, such as skin thinning, stretch marks, and increased susceptibility to infections. If your condition requires extended treatment, your doctor will monitor you closely and may recommend periodic breaks from the medication.

13. Can I use makeup or skincare products while using Neo Medrol?

It's best to avoid applying makeup or other skincare products over areas treated with Neo Medrol, as these products can interfere with its effectiveness or cause further irritation. If you must use makeup, wait until the medication has fully absorbed into the skin, and choose non-comedogenic products to avoid clogging pores.

14. What should I avoid while using Neo Medrol?

While using Neo Medrol, avoid exposing the treated area to harsh chemicals, soaps, or detergents, which can irritate the skin. It's also wise to avoid prolonged sun exposure, as the corticosteroid component can make your skin more sensitive to sunlight.

15. Can Neo Medrol cause an allergic reaction?

Although it's rare, some individuals may experience an allergic reaction to Neo Medrol, especially those allergic to neomycin or other components in the formula. Signs of an allergic reaction include rash, hives, difficulty breathing, or swelling of the face and throat. If any of these symptoms occur, stop using the medication immediately and seek medical help.

16. **Will Neo Medrol interact with other medications?**

Since Neo Medrol is applied topically, the likelihood of drug interactions is lower than with oral medications. However, it's always a good idea to inform your doctor about any other medications, supplements, or herbal remedies you're using to avoid potential interactions, especially if you're using other topical treatments.

17. **What happens if I accidentally get Neo Medrol in my eyes?**

If Neo Medrol accidentally gets into your eyes, rinse them thoroughly with water immediately. While mcdrysone is sometimes used in ophthalmic preparations, the formulation of Neo Medrol is not intended for eye use, and it could irritate. If the irritation persists, contact your doctor.

18. How should I store Neo Medrol?

Store Neo Medrol in a cool, dry place away from direct sunlight and out of reach of children. Make sure the cap is securely tightened after each use to prevent contamination. Do not freeze the medication, and avoid storing it in excessively hot or humid environments, like a bathroom.

19. Can I stop using NeoMedrol once my symptoms improve?

It's important to continue using Neo Medrol for the full duration prescribed by your doctor, even if your symptoms improve early. Stopping the medication prematurely can result in incomplete treatment, leading to a recurrence of the infection or inflammation.

20. What should I do if my symptoms worsen?

If your symptoms worsen or new symptoms appear while using Neo Medrol, stop using the medication and contact your healthcare provider. Worsening symptoms could indicate an allergic reaction, drug resistance, or an underlying condition that requires a different treatment approach.

By understanding the answers to these frequently asked questions, you'll be better prepared to use Neo Medrol safely and effectively. Always consult your doctor or pharmacist for personalized advice based on your specific condition and medical history.

Chapter 7

Storage and Expiry Information

When it comes to medications like Neo Medrol, proper storage is key to maintaining its effectiveness and ensuring it works as intended. Many people overlook how important it is to store medications correctly, but failing to do so can lead to reduced potency or even render the medication completely ineffective. Neo Medrol contains both an antibiotic (neomycin) and a corticosteroid (medrysone), which are sensitive to certain environmental factors. By storing it properly and knowing when it has expired, you can make sure you're getting the best possible results from your treatment.

Proper Storage to Maintain Effectiveness

Medications are typically labeled with storage instructions, but it's common to be unsure about the details. Neo Medrol is no exception—it has specific conditions that help ensure the active ingredients remain stable and effective throughout its shelf life. To get the most out of your Neo Medrol, here are some practical storage tips.

1. Keep Neo Medrol in a Cool, Dry Place

The most critical factor in storing Neo Medrol is temperature. Ideally, the medication should be kept at room temperature, generally between 15°C and 30°C (59°F to 86°F). Extreme temperatures—whether too hot or too cold—can alter the chemical composition of the active ingredients. For example, exposing the ointment to high heat can cause the base to melt or separate, reducing its effectiveness. Cold temperatures, especially freezing, can cause the medication to lose its uniform consistency, making it harder to apply and potentially less effective.

A common mistake is storing medication in the bathroom, where it's exposed to fluctuating temperatures and high humidity due to hot showers or baths. Instead, consider keeping Neo Medrol in a cabinet in a bedroom or hallway, where the environment is more stable. Just make sure it's out of reach of children and pets.

2. **Avoid Direct Sunlight**

Sunlight can degrade the medication, particularly the neomycin and medrysone components. These ingredients can break down when exposed to ultraviolet (UV) light, losing their effectiveness over time. For this reason, it's essential to store Neo Medrol in a drawer, cupboard, or any area away from direct sunlight.

If you're traveling and need to take Neo Medrol with you, ensure it's stored in a shaded part of your luggage or in a toiletry bag that doesn't allow light to penetrate. Similarly, avoid leaving it in hot cars or on windowsills, as these spots can expose the medication to harmful light and fluctuating temperatures.

3. Ensure the Cap is Tightly Closed

Another key aspect of storage is keeping the cap of the Neo Medrol ointment tightly closed after each use. Exposure to air can cause the medication to dry out or change consistency. When air gets into the tube, it can also lead to bacterial contamination, which can make the product less effective or unsafe to use. Make it a habit to close the cap properly after every application and store it upright, if possible, to avoid leakage or air exposure.

4. Be Mindful of the Expiry Date

Like all medications, Neo Medrol comes with an expiration date printed on the packaging. It's important to keep track of this date, as using the ointment beyond its expiration can lead to reduced potency or potential harm. After the expiry date, the active ingredients in the medication may degrade, meaning they won't work as effectively to treat your skin condition. In some cases, expired medications can also cause skin irritation or infection, especially if bacterial contamination has occurred over time.

Signs That the Medication May Have Expired

While the expiration date is the most obvious indicator that it's time to throw out your Neo Medrol, there are also other signs that the medication may have gone bad. Even if the expiry date hasn't passed, improper storage can cause the medication to spoil early. Here are some warning signs to look out for:

5. **Changes in Color or Consistency**

Neo Medrol typically has a smooth, uniform consistency. If you notice that the ointment has become discolored, grainy, or watery, this could indicate that it's no longer safe to use. These changes could be a result of heat exposure or air getting into the tube, both of which can degrade the medication.

Discoloration can also be a sign of bacterial growth, especially if the tube wasn't tightly sealed after use. If the ointment looks or feels different from when you first started using it, it's better to err on the side of caution and dispose of it.

6. **Unusual Smell**

Neo Medrol doesn't have a strong odor, so if you detect a strange or unpleasant smell coming from the tube, it could be a sign that the medication has gone bad. Changes in odor can indicate that the ingredients are breaking down or that bacterial contamination has occurred. In either case, it's best to discard the medication and get a new prescription from your doctor.

7. Skin Reactions

If you begin to notice that your skin is reacting differently to Neo Medrol—such as increased irritation, redness, or itching—this could be a sign that the medication has lost its potency or become contaminated. While these symptoms can also be related to the condition you're treating, an expired or degraded product can cause unexpected reactions. If you suspect the medication isn't working as well as it should, or if your skin starts to react negatively, stop using it and consult your healthcare provider.

8. Disposing of Expired Neo Medrol

When it comes time to dispose of expired Neo Medrol, it's important to do so safely. Do not flush it down the toilet or pour it down the drain, as this can contribute to environmental pollution. Instead, check with your local pharmacy or healthcare provider to see if they offer a medication disposal program. Many pharmacies have designated bins for safe disposal of unused or expired medications.

If a disposal program isn't available in your area, you can mix the medication with an unappealing substance, such as coffee grounds or cat litter, and place it in a sealed plastic bag before throwing it in the trash. This method helps prevent accidental ingestion by children or pets and ensures that the medication won't leach into the soil or water supply.

Storing Neo Medrol properly and keeping an eye out for signs of expiration are simple but important steps to ensure you're using the medication effectively. By following these guidelines, you can maximize the benefits of Neo Medrol and avoid the risks associated with using expired or improperly stored medication.

Conclusion

In concluding our comprehensive guide to Neo Medrol, it's essential to reflect on the multifaceted role this medication plays in treating various skin conditions. Understanding Neo Medrol, from its composition to its proper use, not only empowers patients but also fosters a sense of responsibility in managing their health. This guide aims to illuminate the critical aspects of Neo Medrol, including its application, side effects, precautions, and storage, equipping readers with the knowledge they need to use this medication safely and effectively.

Neo Medrol combines the properties of neomycin, an antibiotic, and medrysone, a corticosteroid, making it particularly effective for treating inflammation and infections of the skin. For many patients, this dual action is a game changer, offering relief from symptoms that can significantly impact quality of life. However, with this effectiveness comes the responsibility to use Neo Medrol correctly. It is vital to adhere to the prescribed dosage and application instructions. Overuse can lead to complications, including skin thinning and increased susceptibility to infections, which is why understanding how to use Neo Medrol safely is so important.

Moreover, awareness of potential side effects can enhance a patient's experience with Neo Medrol. Knowing what to expect allows for better management of any reactions and ensures that patients feel confident in their treatment plan. For instance, while common side effects like localized irritation may be manageable, being alert to more serious reactions can lead to prompt medical attention when necessary. This proactive approach to health care can make a significant difference in treatment outcomes.

The importance of precautions and warnings cannot be overstated. Patients with certain allergies or those who are pregnant should consult with their healthcare provider before using NeoMedrol. By being informed about drug interactions and the specific considerations for sensitive areas of the body, users can avoid complications and promote safer use. Education is empowering, and when patients understand the nuances of their medication, they can participate more actively in their care.

Beyond the immediate use of Neo Medrol, integrating additional lifestyle changes can maximize its benefits. Healthy skin practices, such as maintaining proper hydration and following a balanced diet, can support the healing process. These small but impactful changes can work in tandem with the medication, providing a holistic approach to skin health.

Additionally, it's crucial to keep track of Neo Medrol's expiration date and store it properly. Many people underestimate the importance of medication storage, but it plays a pivotal role in ensuring that the treatment remains effective. Knowing when to dispose of expired medications safely is equally important, helping to prevent unintentional harm and fostering a sustainable approach to health care.

In essence, using Neo Medrol is more than just applying medication; it is about understanding the broader context of skin health and the role that treatment plays in one's overall well-being. The journey of managing skin conditions can often feel overwhelming, but with the right tools, knowledge, and support, patients can navigate this path with confidence.

As we conclude this guide, we encourage readers to continue seeking knowledge about their treatments, engage openly with healthcare providers, and prioritize their health. Every small step taken towards understanding and managing skin conditions leads to more significant strides in achieving better health outcomes. Embracing a proactive approach will not only enhance the effectiveness of Neo Medrol but also contribute to a more empowered and informed experience in managing skin health.